Penis Enlargement

the Easy

Surgery-Free

Way

edited by

Life Science Institute

© 2005 Thompson Publishing

ISBN: 0-9763862-9-1

Contents

Introduction

Recent independent clinical studies reported in scientific journals have demonstrated an amazing fact; significant penis enlargement can be achieved without surgery or special diet.The studies produced outstanding test results like these: all men participating in the studies achieved measurable increases in actual penis size; increases were of length and girth size; put an end to premature ejaculation, give you a prostate gland that will perform for you into your later years and get you ejaculating like a porn star!

In addition, other benefits were reported in the studies: increased fullness and firmness of the penis; spontaneous weight loss; smaller waistline and other positive changes such as increased self-esteem and self-confidence.

If you have ever thought that you would like to have a larger, firmer, fuller penis you owe it to yourself to learn about these easy, step-by-step methods.

There's something very special about knowing that you look and feel your very best. There's a special magic in moving easily, gracefully and feeling great. You will have an opportunity to explore the exciting new evidence for a new, simple method to help you achieve your personal penis development goals.

The methods described in this book can be used with complete confidence since it is a totally natural method of learning to improve your body with normal bodily processes and normal psychological processes. It maximizes your potential for change and improvement.

For years men have had two choices for penis enlargement: surgery or highly advertised gimmicks that are expensive, complicated and sometimes risky procedures and a sure road to disappointment.

Now for the first time there's a method that's so simple, so natural, so safe that men can use it at home and can enjoy the benefits of a larger penis and increased self-confidence.

Most people like to start a project quickly without fully understanding how it works. We suggest that you take a little time first to understand fully how this program works.

Follow the simple, relaxing, and helpful procedures as you learn by doing. The more you practice these procedures, the more beneficial the results are likely to be. Practice does make perfect!

Overview

In the quest for a larger "package" millions of dollars have been spent on worthless and sometimes dangerous methods. And until now, the results have been largely disappointing. Penis pumps are a gimmick and have proven ineffective in increasing long term penis size. Magic "pills" are at most protein and enzyme supplements that simply fatten the whole body and at worst could be contaminated from unsterile manufacturing conditions.

The first important break through in natural penis enlargement is the role of circulation. Let's go back in time to the period in your life when your penis was just beginning to really develop. The developmental stage in a young man's life is a time of hectic physical, bio-chemical and emotional changes. And the demands for increased blood circulation in the developing areas of the body is at a peak. For the penis to grow and develop, proper blood circulation is vital. For it's the blood that brings the essential chemicals and nutrients that stimulate growth.

The body selects and monitors the process of growth and circulation. If certain demands of the body are more important, those needs may be favored and the penis may be neglected. Without the right combination of nutritional and bio-chemical factors the penis may miss this unique opportunity to grow to its maximum potential.

For more than a decade scientists have been teaching people simple learning techniques for improving blood circulation to various parts of the body. These learning procedures are based on more than a decade of studies which demonstrate that individuals can learn to control blood flow, pulse rate, body temperature and many other body functions formerly believed beyond human control.

Until recently, no one ever thought of applying these methods to the improvement of blood circulation to the penis area so that penis size could be increased even years after the normal developmental stage had passed.

Studies have shown that men can increase actual penis size by improving blood circulation to the penis area with simple, relaxing techniques. Consistent use of these methods produced outstanding test results.

The techniques not only increased penis size, but were effective in increasing fullness and firmness of the penis, reduce premature ejaculation and in solving the problem of men who formerly had Erectile Dysfunction.

Other benefits were reported in the studies like the reduction of bulgy waistlines and a variety of positive effects in some other aspect of their lives. In one follow-up study of men who had their penis's enlarged the men reported increased self-esteem, increased self-confidence and feeling happier in all ares of their lives including increased sexual satisfaction.

Program for Penis Enlargement

While the research studies are fascinating from an academic and scientific point of view, it is the potential of their practical application that is unique.

Fundamentally, the procedure involves basic learning processes. It is a psychological program not a medical one. To construct an effective and practical program requires expertise in psychology and an understanding of the nature of the mind/body relationship.

The issue of how the mind affects the body is one of the most fascinating problems in modern psychology. The mind/body relationship has been the focus of countless studies during the last half century. It has been repeatedly demonstrated that individuals can learn to control blood flow, pulse rate, body temperature and many other body functions.

Critical to many of these learning processes is the use of imagery, the visualization of mental pictures in a kind of play-acting scenario which performs on the movie screen of the mind. Its effectiveness is based on the fact that the subconscious mind reacts similarly to both the real experience and the visual imagery experienced in the mind alone.

An example of this is the effects of stress on an individual. The physical effects of a stressful situation, from increased secretions of hormones to other physiological responses are well known. What is interesting is that the physiological changes are produced by the particular individual's perception of and reactions to what precipitates the stress.

Even more significantly, people can produce the same physiological responses without actually being in a stressful situation by just thinking about it. A vivid nightmare can trigger physiological changes in the body. An intense scene in a movie can have the same effect as can thoughts of fear. These are vivid examples of the power of mental pictures. The more vivid and detailed the mental pictures the more pronounced and prolonged is the physiological response.

It is this unique ability of mental processes to produce physiological responses which is at the heart of the recent research on penis enlargement.

The complexities of the mind and the intricacies of the mind/body relationship have been and probably always will be an unending topic for further investigation and study. It is easier to measure the results of the processes then to fully understand how they work.

The prevailing theory of how natural penis enlargement works is that it is the increase in blood circulation in the penis area, produced by the training techniques involved, which stimulates penis growth.

The fascinating thing discovered in the study of these techniques were certain common denominators: all were essentially effortless - that is they used relaxation methods to learn them; all used simple visual imagery of some type.

Th conclusions are exciting.The methods are simple. They are also non-medical. They are not only relaxing but they are enjoyable. They can be achieved without exotic "trance" states. And they work most effectively when employing visual imagery and relaxation.

How it Works

Operationally, visualization utilizes the untapped potentials already in your mind - including how you think and how you imagine things will be. The process of vividly visualizing again and again and again, through the psychological learning techniques used in this book helps to tap these reserves which we already have in our own minds.

The visualizations help you to alter your internalized self-concept or your self-image. It's this internal self-image that acts as a regulator to control your actions and activities. This regulator functions much like a thermostat to keep your performance within limited ranges. Without effective internal regulators most of us really change very little in our lifetimes. And that's one reason why habits seem to be so difficult to break. We continually conform to our own internalized self-image.

For example, if we are overweight, we tend to stay overweight. And if we usually over-eat and eat the wrong kinds of foods, we tend to continue to do this. After all, that's how we see ourselves, that's part of our self-image. And everything that we do will be consistent with that image. Unless you change your self-image it is almost impossible to change your eating habits and to attain a permanent loss in weight. But once you have a achieved a realistic and positive self-image, you can quickly learn to do better.

Visualization works through utilizing effective learning procedures. You see, our minds exercise enormous powers over our lives. We can literally revolutionize our lives by learning to control our thinking. It has been proven time and time again that as individuals we're literally becoming what our self-image suggests. Thoughts tend to become goals. When we recognize that our thoughts do become goals it becomes clear how easy it can be to defeat ourselves. Again you must first learn how to change your concept of yourself in order to actually change. Visual imagery through visual simulation techniques can promote that new self-concept.

However, <u>positive thinking about your body image is not enough</u>. That is why changing our inner motivation and our self-image can best be achieved by psychologically sound learning techniques.

It's clear that improvements in the self-image can be of enormous benefit to any individual. The fact specific images used to increase circulation in the penis area provide the added benefit of helping to improve the self-image may be more than coincidental - they may be mutually supportive processes.

The key to self-improvement is to learn. This is vitally important since both self-image enhancement and improving circulation are concepts that do not respond readily to conventional learning processes. The self-image often seems to be locked in and any attempts to actively change it seem to run into frequent barriers. Overcoming these barriers is a learning process that will lead to self-fulfillment.

Reprogramming Techniques

Progressive Relaxation - The first of these procedures involves learning deep relaxation. Progressive relaxation is an essential key to rapid and effortless learning and to the alteration of our inner drives and motivations.

We recommend that you set aside a quiet period daily for relaxation or meditation time. The typical amount of time to set aside is about 15-20 minutes.

Visualization - A second factor that is extremely important is visualization - using words, pictures and emotions to provide vivid, visual mental pictures of your goal. These mental pictures repeated over and over again, in a relaxed frame of mind, help you create a new self-image, to see yourself in a different way.

They are like a rehearsal for our daily lives - a practice session. Repeated studies have shown that the subconscious mind cannot distinguish between a real experience and one that is vividly imagined in great detail, these mental pictures become a part of our lives and can affect our habits and our internalized self-image.

Reinforcement - the third important factor is reinforcement. After all we've spent most of our life developing our present self-image. Using visualization consistently and following up with reinforcement will enable you to change your self-image.

Each time you follow the techniques described in this book you will be making more and more progress as it becomes easier and easier and more apart of you.

Perceptive feedback - the fourth important factor in perceptive feedback. Feedback is another essential key to learning. Feedback is simply a process of guided learning that emphasizes correct responses.

Put all these factors together and you have the essence of how visualization works. By following the simple learning program for a few minutes a day, you can learn to influence your bodily processes, change your inner motivations and to change your self-image.

Using the Methods

Now that we have discussed the scientific basis for this exciting new penis enlargement method, it's time to learn the simple instructions for using it.

To review what we have learned so far here are the main points:

1) Scientific studies have proven that you can control bodily functions consciously.

2) It works by teaching simple learning procedures which help to increase blood circulation in the penial area and thus stimulate natural, normal penial growth.

3) The methods are mastered through the use of "mental scripts" which employ a four-phase learning program:

   a) Progressive relaxation - to speed the learning process.

   b) Visualization - to facilitate increased blood circulation in the penial area.

   c) Reinforcement - to ensure and maintain rapid learning and retain what has been learned.

   d) Perceptive feedback - to help in monitoring and improving the learning process.

4) The method is amazingly simple to learn.

This last point is the best part of all. Frequently, scientific data and scientific explanation sound complicated. But all one has to do is to read a script, or rehearse it in one's mind, or listen to a recording of it or have someone else read it to you and then follow the simple relaxing suggestions that one thinks about, reads or hears.

Ways of Using the Scripts

The key to the visualization process is the script, for it is the script that is the heart of the learning program. The script utilizes proven learning techniques and the four sequential elements of the method: progressive relaxation, visualization, reinforcement and perceptive feedback. The script teaches the appropriate visualizations that have been shown to increase penis size by improving circulatory processes, while simultaneously enhancing the self-image.

Since the script is essentially a learning program, your goal should be to learn the process in an easy and relaxed manner.

There are four ways the scripts can be learned:

1) The first and most obvious method is to read the appropriate script to yourself. Just sit back in a soft easy chair and read the script slowly and silently to yourself. As you do, follow the suggestions and instructions given in the script - except of course you will be keeping your eyes open for the full reading. Be sure that your are seated comfortably and your are away from all distractions. Each time you read the script you will be reinforcing the learning process.

2) The second method is to study the script thorough-ly until you have learned its basic concepts and then review the complete scripts in your own mind as completely and vividly as possible. Since the process is simply a learning process, this method can be surprisingly effective once you have a thorough understanding of the information the script

and then use it consistently.

3) The third method is to have a friend read the scripts to you in a slow, relaxed, easy-going tone of voice. Some men find it is most effective if the script is read to them by a man others by a woman.

4) The fourth and perhaps the most convenient way is to listen to a recorded version of the script. If your prefer this method we suggest that you read the script first, at least once, and then use recordings for subsequent sessions. This method is highly effective for most because it is a passive, relaxing procedure and because it is very vivid. And it can help many people learn faster and assimilate the learning process more completely. For privacy you may prefer to listen to the recordings with an inexpensive earphone or set of headphones.

To emphasize: you can use any one of the four learning methods described here, or any combination of the four methods. In fact, you may find it beneficial to vary the method that you use occasionally,

Scripts Overview

Script one is called the basic program. It contains all of the ingredients for using the visualization successfully: progressive relaxation, visualization, reinforcement and perceptive feedback. As such it could, if desired, be used exclusively throughout the program. However, the effective utilization of the two additional scripts can help you accelerate your progress, help you to enhance the effectiveness of the program and help you maximize your results.

Script two is the accelerated program. At first glance script two may seem quite similar to script one. However, as you actually begin to use the script, you'll find that the relaxation process is more advanced and the imagery more vivid and intense. The step-up in detail enhances the effectiveness of the learning program. Script two provides additional mental pictures to help expedite the learning process. To accelerate and enhance learning the method, begin alternating scripts one and two every other day any time after week 4.

A third script, called the maximum effects program can be used once or twice a week as an alternate to the other scripts or an extra anytime throughout the entire program. It is especially helpful for insuring rapid progress, overcoming "plateaus", etc.

Keep in mind as you read these scripts that it may seem incredible that visualizations such as those used in the scripts can actually help you improve blood circulation in specific parts of the body, that this finding is now well-corroborated by extensive scientific data. Studies have demonstrated that penis enlargement is almost always achieved by these methods.

As you proceed you will also find it helpful to review your progress. But for now, your next step in getting started is to read the scripts and the instructions.

Basic Program

This program is to assist you in developing yourself and is a simple and effective method. You will find it easy and enjoyable. Just let yourself relax and follow the simple procedures.

First make yourself as comfortable as you can by sitting back in a soft easy chair or by lying comfortably on your back in your bed or on a couch. Take a moment to loosen any tight clothing. Take off your shoes so that you will be totally comfortable. Place your arms in a comfortable and relaxed position and begin to relax the muscles of your whole body. Now, as you begin to relax think carefully about the instructions you are reading or hearing. If you are listening to these instructions, or using them from memory, close your eyes so that you'll be even more relaxed.

While you are relaxed, simply follow the instructions and suggestions that you read or hear or remember. You will find it easy to follow these suggestions and instructions.

As you learn to relax and enjoy these suggestions you will find that you become even more comfortable and have and enjoyable experience. The program is easy and will be natural. It will require no special effort. Just relax and let it happen and the program will work automatically.

Remember, you can be confident that the program works. You will find it is easy if you just let it happen almost by itself. The key words are: let yourself feel comfortable; let yourself relax and enjoy it; you will find it pleasant and easy.

The next few minutes is a time to relax totally. It is a time to let the stresses of the day fade away and let the daily tensions drain away. Your program will help you to feel more refreshed and feel more effective - even more alive and vibrant. As you relax, you will learn automatically to feel more and more comfortable. You will find each time you listen to or read this program and relax, it becomes easier and easier.

You are already learning to relax and feel more comfortable. You have already learned the first lesson without effort as you learn to relax. In time you will learn to relax quickly and effectively with or without the script.

Now as you lie or sit comfortably, you are beginning to learn to relax quickly, easily, and effectively. You will begin to find that you breathe more easily and effortlessly. You can learn to relax easily as you say to yourself the words, " I can relax now and breathe comfortably. This my time to relax." Just thinking these words helps you to relax. You are learning to use these words as your own personal program. You can even reduce these words to simply " relax now" to let you drain the tensions of your body away and enjoy deeper and deeper relaxation. Listening to the recording, or reading this script or just mentally thinking the ideas presented here, helps this process of relaxing and enjoying. So say to yourself, " Just relax now; relax now: relax now". See how it becomes easier and easier and more and more pleasant.

Now you are learning to relax and *feel* comfortable. Good. Let the strains and tensions in your body drain away, slip away. You *feel* more comfortable. Now as your are learning to relax and have pleasant feelings and thoughts, you can enjoy relaxation even more. Just take two long, comfortable breaths and exhale slowly and comfortably. (Pause) Now do this again and *feel* the tension just draining away. (Pause) Now you can visualize or see in your mind's eye, a peaceful, relaxing picture of yourself as you *feel* yourself drifting into a deeper state of relaxation. Now take one more breath, slowly and comfortably. Feel your drifting, care free; see your self drifting, floating, more and more relaxed. Enjoy this feeling. Just drift - comfortable, relaxed, and carefree.

* * *

Begin now to relax all the muscles of your body - to let them become loose and as limp as possible. Let's work with one leg - choose either leg and as you follow your program first tighten the muscles of that leg making the leg feel tight and rigid all over. Keep your leg muscles tight for a moment. (Pause) Now let your leg muscles begin to *relax* from your toes up to your hip.Focus your attention first on your toes letting them *relax* ... then on the muscles of your lower leg, letting them *relax* ... then on the muscles of your thigh, letting them relax. That's good. Now tighten up all the muscles of your leg again, and hold them tight for awhile ... then let them *relax* as before starting with your toes and going up until your leg is quite relaxed. OK, that's fine.

Now tighten up your stomach muscles; hold them that way for a moment. (Pause) Now let your stomach muscles *relax*. It will be easy to relax your stomach muscles if first you tighten your stomach muscles and then *relax* them - letting them go. See how good this feels!

Now do the same thing with your chest muscles.

again it will be easy to relax your chest and breathing muscles if first you tighten them and then relax them - letting them go. Tighten them first, now let them relax. (Pause) Feel the relaxation.

Now focus on your shoulders and your shoulder muscles. Tighten them by pulling your shoulders back; feel how tight they are. Now let the muscles of your shoulder relax. Feel the relaxation in your back. Now stretch your neck and tighten those muscles, again, relax. (Pause)

Now do the same thing with the muscles in your arms from the shoulder right down to your fingertips. First tighten these muscles, making your arms and fingers tight and rigid; now let your muscles from your shoulders right down to your fingertips relax.

Now tighten up your whole face. Hold your face that way for a moment. Tight. Tighter. Now relax all the muscles of your face and feel the comfort in your face. Now you can feel even more relaxed all over.

* * *

Your whole body is relaxing. Relaxation is so pleasant and so comfortable. Let go completely and enjoy it. As you relax your whole body, all tension seems to drain away and you soon find a new sense of comfort and well being. Even your breathing is more relaxed. You begin to feel relaxed all over and a bit drowsy and more and more comfortable. Your whole body is relaxed and your mind is at ease and you feel comfortable. (Pause)

Now you can attain even greater relaxation of your body and your mind. You can use your mind to help you. It's so easy. Just imagine that you are standing at the top of a very pleasant stairway with nice colors and soft carpeting. This will become your 10-step stairway to even more comfort and relaxation. Now in you imagination see yourself walking down this stairway slowly step-by-step and as you walk, take each step in time with the count. An as we count see yourself stepping down with each count step-by-step, walking down to greater comfort and more relaxation.

Step #1, relax. You begin to feel so relaxed and drowsy.

Now step down, #2, and feel more drowsy and relaxed, more comfortable.

Now #3. Getting more drowsy and relaxed.

#4. Getting more and more comfortable and relaxed.

#5 You can feel the soft carpeting and feel more relaxed more comfortable.

#6 Relaxed. Comfortable.

#7 More drowsy, more relaxed, more comfortable.

#8 Getting more relaxed, more comfortable.

#9 Relaxed. comfortable.

#10 So drowsy, so comfortable, so relaxed. your body and your mind are both relaxed.

Now continue to relax, more and more. You feel comfortable and relaxed. As you think clearly and effortlessly of every word, your mind and your body feel more and more relaxed. You are breathing in a more relaxed and comfortable manner. With each breath you take you feel more relaxed, and more comfortable.

You are learning to relax very comfortably. Just continue to relax, rest and to read or listen.

Now we will begin to use mental pictures to help your body become more sensitive and responsive. These pictures will teach your body how to function more effectively.

Image #1

Picture in your mind how your body looked when you were about 12 years of age. Picture what your whole body looked like - your penis, your arms and your legs. Try to see yourself as your body looked. Focus on this mental picture of your body. In your mind's eye you are now 12 years old. You can see your body. You can see your penis. Remember some of the disappointment your felt when you saw your body. Visualization can help change that.

As you look at your picture when you were about 12 years of age and feel how you looked, begin to see your body changing. In your mind begin to see your body developing; developing handsome proportions. See your penis getting longer and firmer. Imagine it happening. Feel the blood coursing into your penis as it begins to grow and develop. As you breathe deeply, feel the energy going into your penis. You can begin to feel your penis actually growing longer, fuller, firmer. Now you can feel your penis pushing outward. As you see your penis growing longer and firmer, you feel a pleasant tightness of the skin over your penis. It is growing, longer, larger.

See how your body is becoming more attractive. As you see and feel your penis developing, you can feel how your waistline begins to feel more trim. As your penis develops, your body proportions change and you begin to feel proud of your body.

Your body is beginning to grow and develop as you would like. It will continue to develop as more blood courses into your penis, as your penis becomes longer, larger and firmer and as your body becomes more attractive.

NOW you picture yourself as you will be by the end of this program. In you mind, visualize yourself as you step out of the shower and stand in front of a full length mirror. See how much longer and larger your penis has become - see how attractive you look with a longer, larger, more attractive penis and a smaller, tighter waistline. See yourself vividly, clearly - with your handsome, improved, attractive proportioned body.

Now you have completed your practice with this picture which we shall call Image #1. It has already initiated the process of physiological change. You have begun to see and to feel how you look with a longer, larger, firmer penis and a slim good looking waist.

Now you can relax even more and your body and your mind can feel comfortable and pleasantly deeply relaxed.

Image #2

And now we can turn to Image #2.

You are learning to relax ever more fully and your

mind is focusing on your penis. And now you can focus all of your attention on your penis. Just imagine now that a warm, most, comfortable towel is being placed on your penis. Feel the warmth penetrating into your skin and into your penis. Feel how comfortable and how relaxing the warmth is. As you feel the warmth in your penis you can begin to feel more blood flowing into your penis, stimulating its growth and vibrancy. As the blood flows into your penis it feels healthier, larger, firmer. You can feel the growth process beginning. Now, focus your attention on the blood pulsating from your heart into your penis. It is a pleasant, comfortable, warm feeling. A pleasant pulsation of blood enlarging your penis. A warm, growing sensation. Your penis is beginning to grow from the inside, to feel fuller, firmer, more attractive. See how comfortable your penis feels and how good you feel about your body development and how much more comfortable it makes you feel.

Your mind will continue to help your blood flow to your penis so that it can continue to grow fuller and larger and firmer.

Image #3

And NOW a third Image picture will assist you even more in developing a longer, larger, fuller and firmer penis.

Imagine yourself with the body you've always dreamed of - and being tremendously proud of every part of your body and especially of your penis. You can feel confident and proud of the attractive penis that you are developing. People will admire your body, the body of a proud and confident man. There is no guilt connected with an attractive body, only confidence and mature pride.

A handsome man is a proud man, a man with an attractive penis is confident man. You will like yourself, even admire yourself, more and more as you see your penis developing and as people respond to your attractive body. It is a good feeling, a relaxed feeling, a feeling of great confidence.

As you think of Image #3 you are in a very deep state of total relaxation. Very comfortable. Very relaxed. And your mind focuses on and remembers the 3 images. Twice daily you will enjoy relaxing for a short period of time and vividly picture the 3 images:

Image #1 - Your penis is growing and enlarging, becoming longer, fuller and firmer, just as they would when a boy grows from 12 years of age and then pictures his perfectly attractive body as yours will be, at the conclusion of your imagery programming with a longer, larger, firmer penis.

Image #2 - A sense of warmth, pulsation and increased blood flow which is helping your penis to grow larger, longer.

and

Image #3 - A feeling of great pride and confidence about your attractive body.

Twice each day, you will enjoy relaxing and setting aside a brief period of time to visualize these 3 images. And you will enjoy reading or listening to this script on a regular basis.

Each time that you read or listen to this script you will enter a deeper, more comfortable stage of relaxation. Each time you read or listen you will find that you relax more quickly. And each time that you say to yourself the words "RELAX NOW" you will be able to relax completely, immediately and will then visualize the 3 images.

This script and the 3 images used consistently will help assure you of achieving your body goals. Your penis will grow larger, longer, firmer, fuller, more attractive and your waistline will become slimmer. Following this program on a regular basis will help you to relax relieve stress and tension and enable your to achieve your body goals.

Practice the imagery technique with the 3 images twice daily and you will enjoy the benefits of a handsome, more attractive body.

Remember these helpful hints:

1) Read the script or listen to the recording on a regular schedule.

2) Twice daily say the words "RELAX NOW" and vividly picture the 3 images.

3) Each time that you do, it will become easier, faster and more automatic.

These hints are your key to larger, firmer, longer penis and a slimmer, trimmer waistline.

And now to conclude this script count to five after which you will feel wide awake, happy and refreshed.

One -feeling good, feeling pleasant, getting up.

Two - More alert, refreshed, enthusiastic.

Three - Stretching your arms and legs and body - feeling good, refreshed.

Four - Eyes wide open, feeling wonderful.

Five - More alert. Feeling good. Feeling refreshed. Feeling vigorous.

Accelerated Program

Script Two:

Now that you've learned the basic features of the program and certain physiological processes have begun to have their effect, it's time to strengthen these processes to achieve maximin results. By simply following the procedures you will find that it's easy to achieve your personal goals and have a attractive body.

Sit back in your soft, easy chair or lie comfortably on your back on your bed or couch and let yourself relax. Take off your shoes and loosen any tight clothing so as to be more comfortable. Place you arms in a comfortable and relaxed position and let your whole body relax. Say to yourself: "Relax now. Relax now." Now as you continue to relax, read or listen to the following instructions. If your are listening to these instructions or following them from memory, close your eyes so that you'll be even more relaxed.

Since you have already learned a great deal about the art of relaxing, it will be easier and easier to relax more quickly and more deeply. You will find that you breathe easily and effortlessly. Keep thinking to your self: "Relax now. This is my time to relax." Just thinking these words helps you to relax more deeply. So relax and let the tensions continue to drain away.

Now we will repeat some of the things we learned before, making them more and more effective. First, take a long, deep breath, hold it for moment - now, exhale slowly, comfortable. (Pause) Feel the relaxation an feel the tension drain away. Now do this over again and while taking a deep breath, visualize in your mind a peaceful relaxing picture of you as you seem to drift in space. An exhale, feel yourself drifting, drifting, drifting. Now take still another deep breath, hold it for a moment, exhale and again see and feel yourself drifting - becoming more relaxed more comfortable. Enjoy the feeling. Just drift and relax, carefree.

* * *

As you relax comfortably, you can learn to relax all the muscles of your body even more than before. Let's work with one leg - choose either leg. First tighten all muscles of this leg. Raise your leg slightly, meanwhile tightening all the muscles of your leg - in your thigh, in your calf and in your toes. Tighten them more and more until your leg is rigid - tighter, tighter, tighter. Keep your whole leg tight and rigid for a moment longer.

Now lower the leg and let it relax from your toes all the way up to your hip. As you relax the muscles of your leg, feel the tension drain out, feel the comfortable feeling in your leg. That's good. Feel the tension drain out. Enjoy this feeling as you rest comfortably for a moment. Now, let's do this again: tightening all the muscles of the same leg, raising the leg slightly, making the leg so rigid, tight, tighter. Hold it for a moment. (Pause) Now, as you lower the leg, relax all the muscles, feel the relaxation, feel the tension drain away, feel your whole body becoming more comfortable and relaxed. Enjoy this feeling as you relax. OK that's fine.

Now we will learn to relax the muscles of our stomach so as to relax our whole body even more. First tighten up the muscles of your stomach by pulling your stomach in more and more. Hold it this way for a moment. Your stomach muscles are now quit tight. Now relax your stomach muscles. Let your stomach expand to its normal position. As your stomach muscles relax, you relax. You feel more comfortable and more relaxed.

Now let's relax our shoulder muscles. First tighten the muscles of your shoulders by pulling your shoulders back, tighter, tighter. Hold them that way for a moment. (Pause) Feel how tight they are. Now, let the shoulder muscles relax. Feel the relaxation in you shoulders. Feel the relaxation spreading to your back. Relax and enjoy this.

Now as you are getting more and more relaxed, let us learn to relax our neck muscles. First tighten your neck muscles by stretching your neck and pulling your head back, until your neck muscles feel quite tight and rigid. Hold them this way for a moment. (Pause) Now let your neck muscles relax and feel how relaxed and comfortable your neck is.

Now let's relax the muscles in one arm - choose either arm. First tighten all the muscles of your arm by stretching your arm and raising it slightly, tightening the muscles in your upper arm, in your forearm, and in your fingers, stretching them out - tighter, tighter, tighter. Keep your arm and fingers tight and rigid for moment. Feel the tightness. (Pause) Now relax your arm and finger muscles as you lower your arm. Feel the comfort and relaxation. Relax and enjoy this feeling.

Now let's relax our facial muscles. First tighten your facial muscles, tightening your mouth, feeling the tightness in your mouth, in your cheeks and in your neck. Hold your face like this for a moment. Now just let your facial muscles relax and feel the warmth and relaxation in your whole face.

Now that your have relaxed many of the muscles of your body, as you relax, see how easily your breathe; how comfortable your whole body feels; how comfortable you feel. Enjoy this wonderful, comfortable feeling. (Pause)

* * *

Now you can relax both your mind and your body. It's so easy. Your mind can help your body and your body can help your mind. Imagine now that you are standing at the top of a very pleasant-looking stairway, a stairway with nice colors and with soft, soft carpeting. See this stairway in your mind's eye. This 10-step stairway will now become your stairway to greater comfort of mind and body. Now in your vivid imagination we shall walk down this stairway to greater comfort and relaxation, step-by-step, slowly and comfortably. Let us step down as we count.

Step down #1 into the the soft carpet and relax.

Now step down #2 and relax even more, getting more comfortable, more relaxed.

Step #3, into the soft carpeting and feeling more and more comfortable.

Step #4 comfortable.

Step #5 getting more and more relaxed.

Step #6 more comfortable, more relaxed.

Step #7 so comfortable, so relaxed.

Step #8, more and more relaxed, more comfortable.

Step #9, relaxed, comfortable.

Step #10, the last step, comfortable, the step to the deepest comfort and the deepest relaxation.

See how both your body and your mind feel completely relaxed. You feel content, sure of yourself, at ease with the world. Just relax and enjoy it. As you read or listen your body will learn to respond effortlessly and function more efficiently and as you continue to relax you will see some pictures in your mind. These pictures will instruct your body how to behave and function - easily, relaxed and without effort.

These pictures will be called bio-images 4, 5 and 6. Like the other images you have been learning, these mental pictures will help your body become more sensitive and responsive and to function more effectively.

Bio-image #4

Picture in your mind this scene; you are lying comfortably on a pleasant, sunny beach. You are by yourself in a beautiful, private, secluded spot. Your eyes are closed and you are relaxing comfortably as you feel the pleasant warmth from the sun. You feel warm, comfortable and pleasant.

As your relax you notice how warm and pleasant your penis feels. You feel the friendly warmth of the sun spreading the sensation of warmth all over your penis.

Your penis begins to tingle and you feel it getting larger, longer, fuller, firmer. Your penis is growing. You can feel it swelling upward toward the sun. You feel it getting larger, longer. Your penis is growing and becoming more and more attractive each day. You enjoy this pleasant feeling of growth. You can sense it growing - you feel it getting larger and you enjoy this pleasant, tingling feeling of warmth and growth as your penis swells and grows to larger, attractive, proportions.

Now, as you relax, enjoying the warmth, your mind drifts back to the time when your penis was just beginning to grow in adolescents. You see in your mind how you looked when you were younger. You remember how you looked when your were younger. You remember how you looked and felt when your were younger. You remember that your body would develop into handsome, attractive proportions. Now as you watch you see your penis starting to grow but this time your penis is growing much larger than it did back then. And as you watch you see the image of your self beginning to change. You see your penis growing longer, larger.

You feel it happening. Your feel the blood flowing into your penis making your penis larger, longer. Your penis is growing and developing attractive proportions. You feel pleased and satisfied with the attractive new growth of your penis.

And now you see a new picture of yourself as you will look at the end of this program. You see how large and full and long your penis has become. You see and feel how attractive you are. Your penis is larger and more attractive. You feel more attractive, more poised, more self-confident. You enjoy the great sense of pride that you feel as you see this handsome new image of yourself. Now as you visualize these mental pictures you continue to enjoy the warmth from the sun. The warmth of the sun feels so good. The sun has helped your penis to grow, and your body to reach attractive new proportions.

Bio-image #5

Now, as you relax, your mind flows to thoughts of the gentle rhythm of your body. You enjoy the smooth, relaxing rhythm of your breathing. With each breath you take your penis begins to swell. You feel your penis swelling, growing. Your penis feels larger, fuller, firmer, longer. With each breath you take you feel your penis is getting larger, longer. The oxygen you breath is traveling your bloodstream into the penial area. You feel the rhythms of your body taking the nourishment and nutrients into your penis, helping it grow.

The rhythm is steady, smooth, like the ticking of a clock ... or the beating of a heart. You sense the gentle, smooth beating of your heart as it directs the blood into your penis. You are now in tune with the rhythm of your heart. You feel the pulsations in your penis, bringing the nutrients, helping them to grow. The gentle, smooth pulsation is helping your penis to grow larger, firmer, longer.

Your penis swells and grows with these gentle rhythms of your body. With each pleasant pulsation the rhythm increases the blood flow to your penis. The gentle, consistent rhythm is causing your penis to grow larger and larger. You are pleased with the sensations and you are pleased with the growth. You feel a sense of pride as your penis is growing to longer, more attractive proportions.

Bio-image #6

And now as you enjoy this comfortable, enjoyable feeling, imagine now that you are seated in front of an elaborate computer that you control. The computer is located deep inside your won mind. You see yourself inside your mind, feeling confident and secure and in control. You are in charge of this computer. You reach forward now and press a button to direct the blood flow into your penis. You follow the direction of your blood. You feel yourself flowing with it as if you were sailing in a smooth boat gliding into your penial area. The smooth and gentle ride takes you into the penial area where you can watch and supervise the growth process.

You see the nutrients going to the cells. You watch the cells grow and expand. You sense each process as the penis increases in size.

And now you sit back and enjoy the warm comfortable sensation of the blood circulation as it goes into the penial area. You imagine a long train carrying extra nutrients and nourishment into your penis and as it does you feel your penis growing. You feel it getting larger and larger. And as your penis becomes more and more attractive you feel a sense of pride in your new, attractive body. Your body has become so much more attractive, so much more handsome. You feel attractive. You feel confident, secure and pleased about your attractive new body.

And each day you will continue to direct the flow of

blood and nutrients into the penial area as your penis continues to grow larger and larger.

Now that you have learned to relax and your mind has helped your body to grow and develop as it should, you will remember to relax daily and employ these three Bio-images daily:

Bio-image #4 - Your penis is growing and enlarging as you enjoy the pleasant feeling of warmth from the sun shining down on you.

Bio-image #5 - You are in tune with the rhythms of your body and you feel the gentle pulsation of blood flowing into your penis.

and

Bio-image #6 - you direct the computer that controls your body to send an extra flow of blood into the penial area. You feel a pleasant sense of pride in your attractive new body.

Each day that you read or listen to this script you will learn to feel more relaxed, more comfortable about yourself, more self-assured. You can use the words "relax now" to help you drain the tensions out of your body and to relax completely.

You have learned to relax and to use the three bio-images to assist your body in performing the functions you need to develop your breasts and your body. You can attain your goal of having an attractive body, one you can be proud of.

Using this program will help you to achieve your

body to function as you would wish, and help you to achieve your goal of an attractive body.

Practice these three Bio-images twice daily to help your mind and your body function as you would wish. Enjoy these practice periods for their relaxation and for the vital growth they are making it possible for you achieve.

And now to conclude this script count to five after which you will feel wide awake, happy, and refreshed.

One - feeling good, feeling pleasant, getting up.

Two - More alert, more refreshed, enthusiastic.

Three - Stretching your arms and legs and your body - feeling good, feeling refreshed.

Four - Eyes wide open, feeling wonderful, feeling vigorous.

Five - More alert, feeling refreshed, feeling vigorous.

Starting On Your Own Personal Program

Now that you understand the basic fundamentals of Bio-imagery programming, and the scientific evidence on which it is based, you can begin your own personal body development program. As you begin, however, it's important for you to be aware of the vital role that attitude plays in your progress on the Program - and in fact, in your successes in almost very aspect of your life.

Here are some important thoughts to keep in mind as you begin your program. Decide to start your new Program now, and EXPECT to succeed. Get excited about your goal - be enthusiastic. Enthusiasm generates persistence. And persistence is important in any self-improvement program. The best self-improvement program in the world means little or nothing to the person who doesn't follow it. So as you begin your program decide to be persistent. Remember that people learn at different rates and that some people respond quickly, while others may respond more slowly. If you're serious about reaching your body development goals you owe it to yourself to give the method a thorough try.

You have nothing to lose by trying - and you have the potential of an attractive body to gain! Follow the program completely and carefully. Keep your goal continually before you. Focus enthusiastically and excitedly on the mental picture of your new, attractive body. Focus on your goal and you'll help make it happen - remember that we always gravitate toward that goal that we think about most.

Concentrate on the rewards of success and not on the fear of failure. When we dwell on the fear of failure we are uncon-sciously bringing failure upon us as our goal.

Imagine and visualize your success in everything you do. See the results of your goal even before you have achieved it, understanding that by changing your self image you can help yourself immensely in many aspects of your life.

As you pursue your goal on this program it's vitally important to understand the difference between persistence and effort. Persistence means merely using the program on a consistent basis. Effort means trying. While trying may be important in many endeavors, it can actually be a hindrance here. In Bio-imagery programming the learning process operates on a different level. You are NOW learning to be aware of different bodily signals. Your new training will be most effective when you literally let go . . . when you just let it happen. *

So focus your enthusiasm on your goal and on stick-ing with the program. If you do, the improvements in your self-image can begin to take place. And each time you use the program the visualizations become more vivid, more intense. As you use the program, put a value on the benefits that can be derived from it. How valuable would it be to have a handsome, sexier body? What could it mean to you in terms of personal pride and self-confidence? The benefits from this program could make it one of the most worthwhile programs you've ever used - rewards far more valuable than the few minutes a day you spend at it.

So decide to start today on your personal body devel-opment goals. Remember that Bio-imagery programming can be your key to the body you've always dreamed of. The important elements are all here: The goal. . . of an attractive body for you. The evidence. . . taken from scientific studies. The technique... embodied in a carefully designed program built with the consultation of experts. And the program. . . designed to help you achieve your goals. Now is the time to begin your personal body enhancement program.

Start today on an exciting new program for improving your body and your self-image. As you use the program, continue your quest to learn as much as you can about the method. Increasing your knowledge of the program can help you to achieve maximum results with it. You may have started the program without reading all the chapters. If so, it is recommended that you now read these chapters which explain Bio-imagery programming and the scientific data in which it is based. Then, as you use the program each day, you'll find that this additional material will make the method more effective as well as more meaningful.

In addition you'll find in the chapters that follow in this book, many additional ideas and suggestions that will help you to maximize your results and enhance the effectiveness of the program.

*Research has shown that individuals who "tried" to learn control of bodily functions through biofeedback methods were having difficulty until they quit trying. Then, when they had literally given up trying, they suddenly discovered that they had learned it almost automatically. Although this program differs from biofeedback (no elaborate equipment is used to learn this program) the same principle applies here: relax and just let it happen. Relaxation is the key to learning; "effort" is contradictory to relaxation.

Improving The Effectiveness of The Program:
How To Achieve Maximum Results

The results of feedback on this program are fascinating. Many men are skeptical, at first, that it can work. After all, it seems so easy. How could something so simple actually increase penis size? Results show that for those who do follow the program to completion, the results are generally very favorable.

Individuals do vary, not only in their motivation to stick to a program, but in the results they achieve. Although scientists may cry for greater accuracy through verified measurements, the enthusiastic men who enjoy the results feel differently.

One of the most fascinating discoveries that comes from analyzing the clinical data is the existence of the proportioning effect. Although all of the clinical studies measured the increases in penis size, only one examined the concurrent reduction in waist size that seems to take place concomitantly. The reduction in the waist size indicates an even greater increase in the actual perceived size of the penis. A very high percentage of those reporting penis increases also reported a corollary decrease in waist size. An analysis of the data seems to indicate that only those who really could benefit from a waist reduction actually reduced waist size - those men who already had small waistlines increased penis size without any reduction in waist size.

Interestingly enough, there seemed to be no significant relationships between either increase or decrease in weight and either penis enlargement or waist reduction - although substantial numbers of the men benefited from the proportioning effect in clinical studies. This finding - the concomitant improved body proportions and the increase in penis size - warrants further study.

Of particular interest is the finding that the program is totally safe. Although thousands of men have used this program, no adverse consequence has been reported. You will find some men who are slow starters and others who are fast starters. Men of very shape and size have used the program.

Maximizing Your Results

Our analysis of the progress of men who have followed the program makes one thing abundantly clear: every man is unique, progresses at his own rate and in his own pattern of change. The probable reasons for this finding are complex. And certainly all of them are not known. Studies of how people learn, and how they relearn, provide insight into some of the factors which influence the learning process.

It seems evident that the self-image plays a vital role in the learning processes involved in Bio-imagery program.

Everything that you can do to help enhance your self-image can help you to progress more effectively with the Program. That is why the technique of visualization can be helpful. We therefore suggest that during the day you focus on the specific concepts you learned from the scripts regarding the visualizations and reinforce the image of yourself that you wish to attain. Picture vividly the new self-image of your attractive, handsome body. Create your own visualizations of leaving your old self-image behind. See yourself walking away from it. Your old self-concept will begin to change as you get closer and closer to your new, improved self-image. And let go of your skepticism. Believe that you can succeed. And know that the program works.

Find other ways to reinforce your new improved self-image. Keep in mind that your self-image is a central factor that helps you to move forward quickly. Most importantly, use the scripts consistently. Know that they were designed by internationally-known consulting psychologists and that the learning procedures that they incorporate are designed to help you enhance your self-image as you use the program.

You may also wish to use a technique for reinforcing your new improved self-image that has been suggested by one of the researchers on this method: find a picture of a man with the kind of body you would like to have and paste over the picture a picture of your own face. From time to time look at this picture as you are visualizing the progress you are making towards your goal.

As you are progressing toward your goal it is also helpful to understand some of the factors which may have inhibited the development of your breasts during your adolescent years. Many men have reported feeling a sense of anxiety, and perhaps undue concern, about the development of their own penis during their developmental stages. In our culture, with its emphasis on youth and virility, this kind of anxiety is not uncommon and it could be a contributing factor in inhibiting the normal development of the penis during the developmental stages of a young boy's life. This type of anxiety may help account for the fact that psychologists have reported case studies in which men enjoyed a natural increase in penis size following psychotherapy.

HOW TO ENHANCE THE
EFFECTIVENESS OF THE PROGRAM

To maximize your success as you begin the program, keep in mind these three important facts:

1. Thousands of people have learned the procedures involved in controlling blood flow for a variety of different purposes.

2. In applying these learning procedures to penis enlargement it's clear that men of every shape, size, and description have learned to enlarge their penis.

3. By following appropriate procedures virtually all men can learn to use this method effectively.

What are the appropriate procedures? One essential factor is being ready to learn. The only thing that can hold you back is the rigidity of your own self-image. A deeply etched self-image can erect subconsciously oriented inhibitions in the learning pathways.

At times it seems that the self-image can provide a passive oppositional aura which acts as a barrier that creates slow starters, causes plateaus, and precipitates other difficulties which interfere with the desired results.

This underscores the importance of the Scripts. As you use your Scripts you will notice the careful emphasis placed on being proud of your body and in feeling good about yourself. All of the terminology throughout the Scripts has been carefully selected to help break through any barriers that might be caused by a poor self-image - and in fact are designed to help you enhance your own self-image. It is important to understand that you cannot exceed the limits set by your own self-image. However, you can improve your self-image and in effect adjust the limits upward.

It is no accident that because the self-image plays such a vital role in this program that so many men report improvements in many other aspects of their lives. In clinical studies, researchers report such diverse benefits as men feeling better about themselves, getting better golf and bowling scores and feeling happier in many other aspects of their lives. These changes seem to be a direct result of the improvement in self-image that takes place with the penis enlargement that occurs.

As you progress on your personal program there are a number of things that you can do to help enhance the effectiveness of the results. For one thing, as we have mentioned, you can work on improving your self-image in many other ways. For example, you can use the visualization techniques throughout your day - as you are walking, standing, sitting, working, etc. Another thing you can do to help is to learn more about your self-image itself.

How to Overcome Plateaus

Your understanding of the role of the self-image in your life can be a great help to you if you should reach a plateau on the program, or are having trouble making a breakthrough. Understand that in all likelihood a setback is nothing more than a temporary barrier. But you can continue to progress by continuing with the program.

If you should reach a plateau you may find it helpful to think about some of the reasons why your subconscious mind may be erecting these temporary barriers. Ask yourself these questions:

1. Do you really want to be an attractive man?

2. If there is something holding you back, what is it?

3. Do you recall ever having been told that you are not attractive?

4. Do you remember learning at some point in your life that you should not feel too proud of yourself ?

5. Do you in some way feel that it's bad to think about having a larger penis - or did you ever get this impression through the words or actions of others when you were growing up?

6. Do you remember feeling anxious or concerned about the development of your body when you were younger?

7. What other shackles from your past could be holding you back?

8. Are you afraid to be more attractive because you fear being with the opposite sex?

*   *   *

Look at some of the other aspects of your life. For example:

1. Have you gone on diets in the past but never quite succeeded?

2. Have you started exercise programs and then dropped them?

3. Have you always wanted to have a "makeover", but have never gotten around to it?

4. Have you thought about taking self-improvement classes, but have never done it?

5. Have you wanted to wear more stylish, more debonair clothes but have found yourself always sticking to older styles and more conservative apparel?

6. Did you start this program but then got "too busy" to complete it?

7. Do you think well of yourself - or are you always putting yourself down, criticizing yourself continually?

In each case, the answers to these questions are, to a large measure, controlled by your self-image. If you find that you haven't done many of the things you would like to do, or find that you have neglected striving for goals you would really like to achieve, look to your self-image as one of the keys to the inhibiting factors holding you back. Then, set up a specific plan to improve and enhance that self-image.

HOW TO ELIMINATE PROCRASTINATION

Another technique that you can use to help clarify in your own mind some of the factors that may cause you to delay using this program is to analyze any possible fears or traits that may be holding you back:

1. Fear of failure - Fear of failure affects people in many endeavors and in this case it could provide a convenient excuse for avoiding or delaying using this program.

2. Fear of success - This is a fear that may surprise you. But many people do fear change. More than that they fear the consequences of change. For example, an individual may be subconsciously anxious about avoiding social contacts and relationships with others. Avoiding using a program like this, or failing to progress on it, provides a convenient way of avoiding becoming more attractive to others. And a self-image which tells you that you are not attractive provides a convenient excuse for avoiding those kinds of relationships.

3. Habit - Some people have simply formed the habit of not changing. They find themselves in a "comfortable rut" and they never really explore or try to experience new things.

4. Procrastination - Procrastination is generally an indication of some inner tension or anxiety. It also serves as a convenient way to avoid activities and relationships with others.

This leads to more anxiety and more inner tension and so the natural result is that it's followed by more delaying and avoiding. The cycle is completed as these actions reinforce a poor self-concept and may even result in a sense of failure or hopelessness.

Any of these factors could cause you to delay using the program, or even inhibit your progress on it, without your even being aware of the real cause of the problem. But if you can identify the cause, and confront it, you'll1 be well on your way to overcoming it.

HOW TO INSURE YOUR SUCCESS ON THE PROGRAM

The fascinating thing about the Bio-imagery programming process is that it inherently provides a way to help overcome most of these obstacles. That's why it's so vitally important to use the program consistently. The benefits of improving your self-image go far beyond the intrinsic benefits of improving your body. And each section of the Script has been carefully designed to help you enhance your self-image.

So make a firm decision right NOW to pursue your own personal program enthusiastically. Let go of your old self-image. Design a new improved self-image that is uniquely your own. In the next chapter you'll find a special Script that's been designed to help you to reach your full potential - not only on the program, but in many other aspects of your life as well. So keep pursuing your goal. . . it's a goal that's well worth working for. And believe that you can reach it. You'll soon find yourself on the way to a lovelier more attractive body. . . and more importantly, a self-image that lets you say "You know, I really do like myself."

The Self-Image Script

Since the self-image plays such a vital role in expediting the learning process, it's helpful to enhance the self-image in every way possible. In this chapter we discuss many helpful techniques that you can use to overcome procrastination, plateaus, and slow starts on the program. In this chapter you will find another useful tool: the Self-image Script.

The Self-image Script is an independent program that can provide benefits with or without the use of the body development program. For enhancing your self-image, improving your effectiveness, or for just getting more out of your life, you can enjoy and benefit from this Script.

But you may also find it helpful to use on occasion as you pursue your body development objectives. Use it to enhance and reinforce the body development Scripts by substituting this Script once or twice a week - or perhaps just as an "extra". You may find it helpful in removing some of the learning barriers that now and then surface from an oppositional self-image. This Script provides an ideal supplementary reinforcement procedure for the basic program. It helps you to focus on body-image and not just on physical attributes.

The relaxation portion of the Script is quite similar to the relaxation portions of Scripts One and Two. However, for your convenience, it is included with this Script to enable you to proceed directly through the Script in proper sequence. But since you've already learned a great deal about the art of relaxing, it is divided into three parts. Start with Part 1 when you wish to follow the complete relaxation portion of the program. Start with parts 2 or 3 if you feel you are a "pro" at relaxing quickly, and you wish to get to the Bio-images in as short a time as possible.

Here are several different ways in which the Self-image Script can be used:

1. Use it to enhance the effectiveness of your body development program.

   A. Substitute the self-image Script once or twice weekly for either the basic or accelerated Scripts or

   B. Use it as an extra once or twice weekly. (If you are learning to relax very quickly you may occasionally omit parts 1 and 2 of this Script and begin with part 3.)

2. Use it as an independent program to help you enhance your self-image and improve your effectiveness at achieving other goals in your life. You'll find that this Script can be beneficial to you long after you have reached your body development goals. To help you enhance your self-image, improve your efficiency and effectiveness, this Script, used independently, can provide life-long benefits.

3. Use Parts 1 and 2 of the Script separately for general relaxation and stress release. This section of the Script stands on its own as a useful and effective relaxation program. You'll find that setting aside a few minutes daily for sheer relaxation can be highly beneficial to you.

. Use parts 1 and 2 as an "open-ended" introduction to personal "goal-setting visualizations" which you create in your own mind. The achievement of any goal begins with a strong visual image which you create in your own mind. Using progressive relaxation as a prelude to these visualizations can help you to reach your goals more easily.

Using the Script in this way is easy. Simply go through parts 1 and 2 of the Script. Then, instead of proceeding through the balance of the Script, create in your own mind mental pictures of the personal goals that you wish to achieve. These visualizations, created while you are in a relaxed frame of mind, can be an important factor in helping you to achieve the goals you have set for yourself.

A Maximum Effect Program

Part one:

This program, is to assist you in improving your self-image and your effectiveness, is a simple and effective method. You will find it easy and enjoyable. Just let yourself relax and follow the simple procedures.

First, make yourself as comfortable as you can by sitting back in a soft easy chair or by lying comfortably on your back in your bed or on a couch. Take a moment to loosen any tight clothing. Take off your shoes so that you will be more comfortable and relaxed. Place your arms alongside your body in a comfortable and relaxed position or fold them over your body, whichever is more comfortable, and begin to relax the muscles of your whole body. Now as you begin to relax, think carefully about the instructions you are reading or hearing.

While you are relaxing, simply follow the instructions and suggestions that you read or hear (or think about from memory). You will find it easy to follow these suggestions and instructions.

As you learn to follow these suggestions you will find that you become even more comfortable and have an enjoyable experience. The program is easy and is quite natural. It requires no special effort. Just relax and let it happen and the program will work automatically. Remember, YOU can be sure the program works so you can be confident. You will find it is easy if you just let it happen almost by itself. The key words are: let yourself feel comfortable; let yourself relax and enjoy it; you will find it pleasant and easy.

The next few minutes is a time to learn to relax total-ly. It is a time to let the stresses of the day fade away and let the daily tensions drain away. Your Program will help you to feel more refreshed and feel more effective even more alive and vibrant. As you relax you will learn automatically to feel more and more comfortable. You will find that each time you listen to or read this program and relax, it becomes easier and easier.

You are already learning to relax and feel more com-fortable. You have already learned the first lesson without effort as you learn to relax. In time you will learn to relax quickly and effectively with or without the Script.

Now, as you lie or sit comfortably, you will begin to find that you breathe more easily and effortlessly. You can learn to relax easily as you say to yourself the words, "I can relax now and breathe comfortably. This is my time to "relax." Just thinking these words helps you to relax. You are learning to use these words as your own personal program. You can even reduce these words to simply "relax now" to let you drain away the tensions of your body and enjoy deep-er and deeper relaxation. Listening to the recording or read-ing this script, or just mentally thinking about the ideas pre-sented here, helps this process of relaxing and enjoying. So say to yourself, as you do: "Just RELAX NOW; RELAX, NOW; RELAX NOW." See how it becomes easier and easier and more and more pleasant.

Now you are learning to relax and feel comfortable. Good. Let the strain and tensions in your body drain way, slip away. You feel more comfortable.

Now as YOU are learning to relax and have pleasant

feelings you can enjoy relaxation even more. Just take a long, comfortable breath and exhale slowly, and comfortably. (PAUSE) Now do this again and feel the tension draining away. (PAUSE) Now visualize or see in your mind's eye, a peaceful, relaxing picture of yourself as you feel yourself drifting into a deeper state of relaxation. Now take one more breath, slowly and comfortably. Feel yourself drifting, care-free; see yourself drifting, floating, more and more relaxed. Enjoy this feeling. Just drift comfortable, relaxed, and care-free.

PART 2:

Begin now to relax all the muscles of your body letting them become as loose and as limp as possible. Let's work with one leg first. Choose either leg and tighten the muscles of that leg - making the leg feel tight and rigid all over. Keep your leg muscles tight for a while. (PAUSE) Now let your leg muscles begin to relax from your toes up to your hip. Focus your attention first on your toes, letting them relax. . . then focus on the muscles in your lower leg, letting them relax. . . then focus on the muscles in your thigh, letting them relax. That's good. Now tighten up all the muscles of your leg again, and hold them tight for a while. . . then let them relax just as before, starting with your toes and going up the leg until your whole leg is quite relaxed. As you relax the muscles of your leg, feel the tensions drain away. Enjoy this feeling as you rest comfortably for a moment. OK, that's fine.

NOW, tighten up your stomach muscles; pull your stomach in tight, hold your stomach that way for a few moments. Feel how tight your stomach is. (PAUSE) Now let your stomach muscles relax. As your stomach muscles relax, you relax, you feel comfortable and more relaxed. See how good this feels!

Now do the same thing with your chest and breathing muscles - by breathing in and holding your chest tight. Tighten the chest muscles first. Then let them relax and let the air out of your lungs. (PAUSE) Do this again, and feel the relaxation.

Now focus on your shoulders and your shoulder muscles. Tighten them by pulling your shoulders back; feel how tight they are. Now, let the muscles of your shoulders relax. Feel the relaxation in your back.

Now stretch your neck by pushing your head up and tighten your neck muscles. Again, hold your head this way for a moment. Now relax your neck muscles. See how good this feels.

Now do the same thing with the muscles in your arms from the shoulders right down to your fingertips. First, tighten these muscles, stretching your arms and fingers and tightening your muscles making them rigid; hold your muscles in your arms tight, even tighter for a while. Now, let your muscles from your shoulders right down to your fingertips relax. Do this again and see, once more, how relaxing this can be.

Now, tighten up your whole face. Tighten the muscles of your mouth, your chin, your cheeks, and your forehead. Hold your face that way for a few moments. Tight. Tighter. Now relax all the muscles of your face and feel the tensions in your face drain away. Feel the comfort in your face. Now do this again. First tightening your facial muscles, then holding them for a few moments, then letting your whole face relax. Now you can feel even more relaxed all over.

Penis Enlargement the Easy Surgery-Free Way

PART 3:

Your whole body is relaxing. Relaxation is so pleasant and comfortable. Let go completely and enjoy it. As you relax your whole body, all tension seems to drain away and you find a new sense of comfort and well-being. Even your breathing is more relaxed. You begin to feel relaxed all over, and more and more comfortable. Your whole body is relaxed, and your mind is at ease and clear and you feel comfortable.

Now you can attain even greater relaxation of your body and your mind. You can use your mind to help you. It's so easy. Just imagine that you are standing at the top of a very pleasant stairway with nice colors and soft carpeting. This will become your 10-step stairway to even more comfort and relaxation. Now, in your imagination see yourself walking down this stairway, slowly, step-by-step, and as you walk take each step in time with the count. And as we count, see yourself stepping down with each count, step-by-step, walking down to greater comfort and more relaxation.

Step # 1, relax. You begin to feel so relaxed and drowsy.

Now step down, #2, and feel more drowsy and relaxed, more comfortable.

Now #3, getting more drowsy and relaxed.

#4. Getting more and more comfortable and relaxed.

#5. You can feel the soft carpeting and feel more relaxed, more comfortable.

#6. Relaxed. Comfortable.

#7.More drowsy, more relaxed, more comfortable.

#8.Getting more relaxed, more comfortable.

#9 Relaxed. Comfortable.

10. So drowsy, so comfortable, so relaxed. Your body and your mind are both relaxed.

Now continue to relax, more and more. You feel :comfortable and relaxed. As you think effortlessly of every word, your mind and your body feel more and more relaxed. You are breathing in a more relaxed and comfortable manner. With each breath you take you find that you are becoming more relaxed, alert, and more comfortable.

You are learning to relax very comfortably. Just continue to relax, rest, and to read or listen.

Now that you have learned to relax, you have already taken the first important step to enhancing your self-image and improving your effectiveness. Relaxation is the foundation for learning to enhance your self-image. It is important to understand that almost all people who fail are anxious and tense - even though they may try to hide this from themselves and from others by pretending that they are happy and carefree.

As you relax, you can accept the fact that some things in your past life added to your insecurity and lack of self-confidence. A basic cause of this insecurity is your poor self-concept - your poor self-image. But now that you understand that, you can change your self-concept. With the help of this Script, and in your self-concept. With the help of this Script, and in a relaxed frame of mind, you can become a winner, and gain self-confidence and find that you have less need - less compulsion to delay and avoid goal achieving activities. You will find that you can improve your effectiveness, enjoy life more, and gain self-confidence. You will find that you can enjoy being decisive, and active, and accomplishing your goals and gaining self-confidence.

As you continue to relax, ask yourself "Why have I lacked self-confidence?" "What has made me feel insecure in the past?" There are only a few basic reasons for this. You may have been fearful that you would not be liked, or would be criticized. Or you may have been afraid that you would be a failure. You might be afraid of success and the independence it brings. Or you may have been anxious about your relationships with other people. Such things lead to anxiety, to inner tension, and so to insecurity and lack of self-confidence. It can even lead to a sense of failure or hopelessness.

But, now you are changing all of that. As you relax, and the tension drains away, you can begin the process of internalizing a good, healthy self-image. Each time you follow this program, you will automaticalLy improve your self-concept, lose tension, and gain self-confidence. You will begin to see that you have a lot to offer, that you are worthwhile, that - as you accept yourself more and more - other people will also accept you more and more and like you more and more. You begin to feel that you are basically good and desirable and capable. And as you gain self-confidence, your inner tensions slip away, and you feel good about yourself - and you can live as you should live, enjoyably and effectively - without tension, and without guilt.

It is important to remember that, like all other people, you will sometimes make mistakes. But like all other people, you are good, you are worthwhile, and you can profit from mistakes, and with increasing self-confidence feel more self-assured, feel more secure, and succeed in reaching your goal of being an effective, happy, attractive person - efficient, decisive, and goal achieving. .

BIO-IMAGE #1:

Now, as you internalize these thoughts in a relaxed comfortable manner, and as you keep on gaining self-confidence and inner security, you can begin to visualize how YOU will look, feel, and act in all social situations. We shall call this visualization Bio-image # 1. Imagine, in your mind, that you are in a social situation with a few people around you. Picture this scene in your mind. See it vividly, in every detail. You are listening to them as they talk. You listen in a relaxed manner, feeling secure, comfortable, and self-assured. Then, when you are ready, you say something to your friends in response to what they have been talking about. You say this easily, comfortably and with complete self-assurance. As you speak, you show how self-assured you are, how you like yourself, and how you know you are also liked. Your friends look at this new you with surprise and delight. They envy you. They admire you. And now you realize that you are likeable for what you are - for the real you. You literally eat up their admiration, their liking for you, and you feel deeply that you are likeable and have much to offer. Your inner security increases, your inner tensions dissolve, and you feel great! You have begun to internalize an improved self-image.

Remember that each time you follow this Script you

will see and feel this mental picture more and more vividly; you will see the new you emerging, the new self-confident, self-assured you: a likeable, attractive, self-assured person. Bio-image # 1 will help you to gain increasing self-confidence each time you visualize it and help you drain away unnecessary anxiety and guilt about yourself.

Now, as you continue to relax we will go on to some other mental pictures that will teach your body how to function more effectively.

BIO-IMAGE #2:

Here is Bio-image #2. Imagine now that you are looking at some photographs, and you come upon a picture of an extremely attractive person with ideal body and look. You now look at this picture more closely. Suddenly, you realize that this is the real you. You look at the picture even more closely. Yes, it is you. You see this new you very clearly. You see a very attractive person who looks and feels poised and self-assured. You look terrific! You study the picture in greater detail. You admire how energetic and happy you look. You become more and more excited as you look at this picture of you.

You look great - in excellent physical condition - healthy and self-assured. You feel how attractive you are. You feel good physically all over. You notice how well-dressed you are and how happy, relaxed, and calm and worry-free you are. Your eyes seem sparkling and smiling. You are smiling pleasantly. You feel vibrant, glowing with health and energy.

As you continue to look at this mental picture, you

can feel yourself becoming more attractive - and getting more and more like the picture. You feel proud of yourself.

Now you can picture yourself as you will be by the end of this program - confident, self-assured, and effective. Just like the photograph. In your mind visualize yourself you stand in front of a full length mirror. See how attractive you look and feel. See how great you look. See yourself vividly, clearly - with your handsomely improved, self-confident manner. You have now enhanced the process of self-image improvement. You have begun to see how you can really look and feel. Now you can relax even more and your body and your mind feel comfortable, and pleasantly, deeply relaxed.

BIO-IMAGE #3:

And now we can turn to Bio-image #3. You are relaxing even more fully now. As you relax picture in your mind a giant movie screen. As you watch, the movie begins, and you see that the same slender, attractive you that you saw in the photograph is the star. You are the star and the director of this film.

As the scene opens the camera focuses on you as you begin your day. You expect another great day. You are smiling and feel a deep down sense of joy and exhilaration as you look forward to an enjoyable day. You feel a sense of optimism and enthusiasm and positive expectancy as you start another great day. You see and feel how great you look - how energetic and healthy and happy you look - and how easily and smoothly and gracefully you move with your trim, well-proportioned, attractive body.

You arc now living the part of the role. It is you and you see and feel yourself in every scene; the major scenes in the movie show you enjoying a full and rich, happy life filled with interesting and exciting things to do. As you go through the day you notice how calm and worry-free you are. You notice how things don't seem to bother or upset you. You handle your life with secure, mature confidence.

You see yourself having fun, enjoying your life and life's activities. Your life is occupied with interesting and exciting things to do. You see yourself enjoying your work and your many social activities, personal relationships, and hobbies. Your work activities are efficient and effective. You are meeting new people and forming new friendships. As you meet other people they are impressed with how friendly and nice you are. As you become a part of the movie you actually feel, as you live and experience the part, the positive emotions that are part of your improved self-image. You feel a reassuring sense of self-confidence. You feel assured and secure. You have pride in your life and your life's activities. And you feel a sense of optimism and enthusiasm.

You feel that this is the real you now controlling your own life and your own activities. You know and feel how worth while you are and how much you deserve to succeed, to be happy, and to achieve your goals. You see yourself as you do things promptly. You see and feel how decisive you are - reaching decisions promptly and wisely and then acting on them right away.

And as you feel the positive, happy feelings, you feel the negative feelings you used to have disappearing - like being erased from a blackboard. You feel leaving you the fears of failure, fears of criticism, fears of success and independence, fears of decisions- all the fears that you used to have. You feel leaving you negative procrastinating habits, fears of social and personal relationships and commitments. You feel these and other negative and other self-defeating notions leaving you. You watch as they disappear from the blackboard and you feel a sense of elation and joy and exhilaration and freedom as they leave you.

You watch as they disappear just as if they were in helium filled balloons floating away out of sight in the sky. They leave to make room for a new life of freedom for the real you, the new you. Their place is filled with positive self-expectancy, enthusiasm, optimism, joy and happiness and positive self-esteem and self-confidence.

You feel great as feelings of joy, happiness, excitement, energy, and creativity dominate your mind. YOU feel good about yourself and know how you desire to succeed and how you deserve to succeed. You feel a sense of freedom at being able to control and direct your life. YOU enjoy your new independence and feel a sense of pride in the new you, the real you.

BIO-IMAGE #4:

And now a fourth Bio-imagery picture will assist you even more in enjoying a sense of self-confidence, happiness, and effectiveness.

See yourself in your own mind looking the way you've always dreamed of and feeling tremendously proud of yourself and your life. You feel confident and proud of the way you look. People admire your appearance and they admire you. You have no guilt about being attractive only confidence and mature pride.

With an attractive defiance you feel proud and confident. You like yourself, and others like you. You feel secure and self-assured. You are very pleased with yourself and the way you look. Everything seems right. You look radiantly happy, confident, and proud. You feel pleased that others are friendly to you and admire you.

You are delighted at how well you feel as you move so gracefully and easily. You feel great about your new self-confidence. And every day you feel better and better about yourself.

As you visualize Bio-image #4 you are in a very deep state of total relaxation. Very comfortable. Very relaxed. And your mind focuses on, and remembers the four Bio-images. Twice daily you will enjoy relaxing for a short period of time and vividly picture the four Bio-images.

Bio-Image #1 - Visualize the self-confidence and inner security that you feel and show in all social situations. Feel how self-assured, likeable, and attractive you have become.

Bio-Image #2 - See a photograph of how attractive and self-assured you look. See how terrific you look at the end of this program.

Bio-Image #3 - See a movie of the new you enjoying your life and your life's activities.

Bio-Image #4 - Enjoy a feeling of great pride about your confident and attractive appearance.

Twice each day, you will enjoy relaxing and setting a side a brief period of time to visualize these Bio-images. And you will enjoy following this Script on a regular basis.

Each time that you read or listen to this Script you will enter a deeper, more comfortable stage of relaxation. Each time you read or listen you will find that you relax more quickly. And each time that you say to yourself the words "RELAX NOW" you will be able to relax completely, immediately, and will then visualize the 4 Bio-images.

This Script, and the 4 Bio-Images, used consistently, will assure you of achieving your self-improvement goals. You will become more attractive and YOU will look and feel great. Following this program on a regular basis will help you to relax, relieve stress and tension, and enable you to achieve your self-improvement goals.

And now, to conclude this Script, count to 5 and you will feel wide awake, happy, and refreshed.

1. Feeling good, feeling pleasant, getting up.

2. More alert, refreshed, enthusiastic.

3. Stretching your arms and legs and body - feeling good, refreshed.

4. Eyes wide open, feeling wonderful.

5. More alert, feeling refreshed, and vigorous.

Questions and Answers About the Method

From time to time as you are using this program you may have questions about the method itself, the results it can achieve, or specific questions about its use. This chapter provides a summary of the most commonly asked questions about the program.

Q. What is this new method?

A. It's a simple, effective way to increase penis size in the same natural way that the penis first began to develop in early adolescence.

Q. How does it work?

A. It works by simply improving circulation in the penis area. Proper circulation is vital for the growth of any part of the body because it's the blood that brings the nutrients essential for growth.

Q. How was it discovered?

A. Thousands of people have already learned how to improve circulation for a variety of purposes, and they use these simple methods every day. For more than a decade scientists have been showing people how easily they can use these proven methods at home. But until recently, no one ever thought to see if improving circulation in the penis area would increase penis size in men of virtually any age (even years after the developmental stage had passed). Then, some independent teams of researchers and medical doctors, working separately in different parts of the country, conducted the clinical studies which signaled this exciting scientific breakthrough.

Q. What were the results of these studies?

A. All men participating in the studies achieved measurable increases in actual penis size.

Q. Does this method help reduce mentally induced erectile dysfunction?

Yes, in most cases. One of the studies stated that most of the men in the study reported that they significantly increased their ability to obtain and maintain a full and hard erection.

Q. Are there other benefits from this technique that were reported in the studies?

A. Several. For example, one finding stated that the men in the study who previously experienced high incidences of premature ejaculation reduced or completely eliminated the occurrences during sexual intercourse. In another study men reported the reduction of bulgy waistlines in addition to the increase in penis size. Other studies on penis enlargement indicate that positive changes can occur in many other aspects of life including improved self-esteem and self confidence, as well as improved interpersonal and marital relationships.

Q. Is the technique difficult to learn?

A. It's amazingly simple! It can be learned in the privacy of your own home in just a few minutes a day.

Q. Is it safe?

A. Totally. It is not an artificial program. It's designed to help you to reinstate the natural increases in penis size that began in your early adolescence.

Q. Does it involve physical exercise?

A. No. The fact is that exercise cannot help you increase the actual size of your penis for a very simple reason - the penis contain no muscle tissue. This new method requires no physical effort of any kind - in fact you use it while you are resting.

Q. Does it use any of the pumps, pills or protein/enzyme supplements I've seen advertised?

A. No. These products are designed to help you gain weight on the assumption that some of that weight will be in your penis. Unfortunately, excess weight will go to other parts of the body not your penis.

Q. Obviously, this new method does not involve surgery.

A. That is correct. Prior to the publication in scientific journals of the results of the clinical studies for this new method, surgery was the only other penis enlargement procedure with clinical evidence for its effectiveness. Other methods, some very heavily advertised, have been unable to cite actual studies on which their procedures or products are based.

Q. Are there disadvantages to surgery?

A. Yes. In addition to the expense of the procedure, there are the disadvantages of possible scarring, the possibility of unnatural looking results, the discomfort and the dangers from the anesthetics and possible infections. Complication rates as high as 60 percent have been reported for penis enlargement surgery.

Q. What are the advantages of the new method?

A. It's safe. It's easy-to-use. It's economical. It's natural. And it can be used in the privacy of your own home in just a few minutes a day by men of virtually any age. Best of all it really works.

Q. How long does it take each day?

A. Just a few minutes a day while you're learning the method. After it's learned it can take as little as 1 or 2 minutes a day.

Q. How long does it take to begin to see results?

A. Typically within 2 to 3 weeks. (Occasionally, some cases show results a little later.) Then the increases can continue for up to 12 weeks or more.

Q. When will I have my greatest progress?

A. Although individuals vary, most men seem to enjoy their greatest increases in the second month of the program.

Q. Is any special time of the day preferable for using the

program?

A. The best time is simply the time that's most convenient for you. However, a set time each day has the advantage of helping you form the habit of sticking to the program.

Q. What if I miss a day?

A. Just get back on the program the next day. The program has adequate leeway built in for occasional variations. But if an attractive body is really important to you, keep after your goal.

Q. I would like to reach my goal in less than 12 weeks. Is this possible?

A. Some people do. But it's important to be realistic. The original growth of your penis during adolescence took much longer than 12 weeks. Since you really want to reach your goal, persist in your endeavors and follow the full program.

Q. Is age a factor?

A. Apparently not, at least within the wide age limits that have been studied. In one of the studies the ages of the men ranged as high as 54 years.

Q. How much can be gained?

A. Individual results are dependent on your persistence with following the program. The old saying "you get what you pay for" can be translated into "you get what you are willing to put into it" If you follow the program's instructions persistently you will exceed in shaping the body you dream of.

Q. What if I want further gains later, can I repeat the program?

A. Yes. One of the researchers recommends that after you complete your program that you wait for 3 months and then repeat the entire program again. He reports that the gains con -tinue in the second phase.

Q. I am planning a diet. Can I go on it and still use the program?

A. Yes.

Q. I have tried other methods and they didn't work for me. Why is that?

A. Quite honestly, the only effective methods of penis enlargement, confirmed by scientific research, are this method and surgery
.
Q. I wish to gain just a small increase. Can I limit the amount of increase?

A. Yes. Just use the program until you have reached your goal and then discontinue it.

Q. My waist is already very small. Can I increase penis size without reducing my waistline?

A. Yes. The results indicate that waist reduction typically takes place only for those men who would benefit from a reduction.

Q. Once I reach my goal will my penis remain at its new

larger size?

A. Yes. Although the program includes a simple reinforcement technique that you may wish to use on occasion, professionals using the method report that they have generally found this unnecessary

Q. I once tried a pumping device and my penis became sore and discolored for awhile. Will this happen with this program?

A. No. Since there is no external devices involved in this program you will risk damaging your penis. Instead you will benefit from a proportioning effect which enlarges the penis and reduces the waistline area.

Q. How many inches will I gain?

A. Each individual is unique and results vary from person to person.

Q. Can the Program be used while following a diet and exercise program?

A. You'll enjoy a natural increase in blood flow to the penis when following a healthy diet and exercise regiment. You should ask your doctor if you have any questions regarding the use of the program during these times.

Q. What if I get off to a slow start?

A. Give it a fair try. Many men who enjoyed excellent results with the program were slow starter:

Q. If I fall asleep while I am using the method will it still be effective?

A. It is most effective when you are totally relaxed but alert. It you try to read the Script, rehearse it in your mind, or listen to it when you are overly-tired you may become so relaxed that you fall asleep.

If you find that you do, you can form the habit of remaining alert, although totally relaxed by (1) using the Program when you are reasonably refreshed, (2) sitting instead of lying down (keep your head up instead of leaning it back), and (3) setting one or more timers or buzzers next to you and have them go off at the approximate time you have been dozing off. You'll find that you will quickly learn to become totally relaxed while you continue thinking about the thoughts and images presented in the Scripts.

Q. I feel I have really mastered the relaxation portion of the Scripts and have learned to relax totally. Can I now shorten the relaxation section of the Script?

A. After you have begun to achieve positive results on the program you may shorten the relaxation section of the program as follows: use the full Script one day; then, the next day start your program just prior to the section on muscle relaxation; then, the third day start it just prior to the relaxation segment (the approximate segment is close enough - it is not necessary to be exact).

You may continue to alternate the starting point of the Script on this schedule as long as you feel that you are relaxing as effectively with the shorter relaxation time period - and as long as you continue to get positive results from the program. For maximum benefit from the program, however, you will find it helpful to use the complete program periodically. This will help reinforce the learning process.

Q. Will exercise help?

A. Exercise is beneficial for many reasons - including your waistline measurement which, of course, affects the appearance of your penis. It will not, however, increase actual penis size as this program can.

Q. Are there reasons why my penis did not grow as large as it could have when I was younger?

A. There could be many reasons. The developmental stages of a young boy's life are periods of hectic physical, biochemical, and emotional change. The demands on the body are at a peak.

Q. I've seen other similar programs advertised. Are they any good?

A. That depends totally on the expertise of the person developing the program. You should be certain that any program you use is designed by knowledgeable experts.

The questions and answers in this chapter are the result of extensive experience with the program. Used in conjunction with the rest of the book, the essential information that you need to reach your goal is here for you to transpose into a realistic and handsome body development program.

Our journey, which began with an introduction to a

new penis enlargement discovery, and took us on an interesting voyage through the scientific and practical aspects of the program, now leads us to one inescapable conclusion: while the tour itself may be fascinating, it's the destination which is really far more important.

It's the goal of an attractive body that, in the final analysis, is far more meaningful to you than all of the studies and all of the scientific data. The exciting thing is that now that goal can be transcribed into reality! Now an attractive body is within your reach. And every essential fact that you need to know to insure your success is here.

This book is your road map to that success. Follow it. Use it. Stick with it consistently. Make your journey to an attractive body a delightful and enjoyable experience. Success is within your reach.

Exploring the Scientific
Data for the Method

The learning procedures integrated in the Bio-imagery programming process are based on and enlarge upon, the results of actual studies conducted by scientific researchers and by medical doctors conducting separate clinical tests.

If more than a decade of scientific studies on learning procedures and related processes have demonstrated that individuals can alter bodily functions and processes formerly believed beyond human control. Bio-Imagery Programming is based on sound scientific data.

The entire program of relaxation and habit-training methods used in Bio-Imagery Programming is designed to encourage natural development of the penis and secondary improvement in self-assurance and self-respect. The procedures integrate the findings of psychological research and clinical practice, utilizing natural, psychological methods to improve circulatory processes as a means of improving penis development and enhancing the self-image.

The Bio-Imagery Programming process is based on the general and specific findings from the psychological fields of: learning theory; methods of inducing relaxation so as induce more effective and harmonious general bodily processes; methods of insuring improvement in self-image and self-concept; psychological methods of learning feedback; methods of improved visualization and self-imagery; and the specific studies on the effects of some of these procedures, in both research studies under controlled conditions and in clinical studies under the supervision of qualified professionals.

These studies demonstrate the effectiveness of these methods in improving general physiological functioning and specific and improved circulatory processes which assist in normal development of the penis which may have been inhibited by such factors as: undue tension; inability to focus on one's own natural bodily processes; inability to maintain relaxed concentration; and inhibition in normal learning processes.

It should be noted that none of these methods employs medical devices or techniques, none utilizes the ingestion of any product, and none offers any medical advice or suggestion. Instead the methods are based on learning processes - they are strictly psychological and are presented so as to encourage more effective and more natural bodily processes through time and research-tested psychological principles and methods.

The approach and methods used in Bio-imagery Programming are based on hundreds of studies and experiments, some of them specifically directed to investigating possibilities for improving body-image and to gaining enlargement of the penis.

Over the years it has been learned that people can change not only their behavior and personality, but also their physiological processes, bodily functions, and bodily structure to gain better self-concepts and more effective body-functions. Such methods were used in ancient times but their more recent use is based on learning studies, studies in psychology and especially studies on developmental and learning processes. Many theories have been developed to explain the findings from these studies but no one theory can do justice to all of the findings.

Bio-Imagery Programming is based on these scientific findings and integrates them into a manageable, practical method, so that thousands more can take advantage of the new knowledge. We cannot attempt to provide a comprehensive listing of all of the relevant studies and books used on these studies. Several of the scientific studies have demonstrated the significant and remarkable results which can be achieved using these psychological procedures.

The relevant independent clinical studies were conducted by research scientists and reported in highly respected scientific journals found in most major universities.

www.ingramcontent.com/pod-product-compliance
Lightning Source LLC
Chambersburg PA
CBHW022126280326
41933CB00007B/559